HEALING THE GUT, HEALING THE MIND

The Revolutionary Connection between Gut Health, Nutrition, and Mental Wellbeing

JAMES HALEN

Contents

GUT AND PSYCOLOGY SYNDROME

The GAPS diet is a strict elimination diet that requires its followers to cut out:

• Grains

• Pasteurized dairy

• Starchy vegetables

• Refined carbs

It's promoted as a natural treatment for people with conditions that affect the brain, such as autism.

However, it's a controversial therapy that doctors, scientists and nutrition professionals have widely criticized for its restrictive regimen.

The contents of this book explore the features of the GAPS dietary protocol and examines whether there's any evidence behind its purported health benefits.

WHAT IS THE GAPS DIET AND WHO IS IT FOR?

GAPS stands for Gut and Psychology Syndrome. It's a term that Dr. Natasha Campbell-McBride, who also designed the GAPS diet, invented.

Her theory is that a leaky gut causes many conditions that affect your brain. Leaky gut syndrome is the term used to describe an increase in the permeability of the gut wall.

The GAPS theory is that a leaky gut allows chemicals and bacteria from your food and environment to enter your blood when they wouldn't normally do so.

It claims that once these foreign substances enter your blood, they can affect your brain's function and development, causing "brain fog" and conditions like autism.

The GAPS protocol is designed to heal the gut, preventing toxins from entering the blood stream and lowering "toxicity" in the body.

However, it isn't clear if or how leaky gut plays a role in the development of diseases.

In her book, Dr. Campbell-McBride states that the GAPS dietary protocol cured her first child of autism. She now widely promotes the diet as a natural cure for many psychiatric and neurological conditions, including:

- Autism
- ADD and ADHD
- Dyspraxia
- Dyslexia
- Depression
- Schizophrenia
- Tourette's syndrome

- Bipolar disorder
- Obsessive-compulsive disorder (OCD)
- Eating disorders
- Gout
- Childhood bed-wetting

The diet is most often used for children, especially those who have a health condition that mainstream medicine may not fully understand yet, such as autism.

The diet also claims to help children who have a food intolerance or allergy.

Following the GAPS diet can be a years-long process. It requires you to cut out all foods Dr. Campbell-McBride thinks contribute to a leaky gut. This includes all grains, pasteurized dairy, starchy vegetables and refined carbs.

The GAPS protocol stages

The GAPS protocol is made up of three main stages:

- The GAPS introduction diet
- The full GAPS
- A reintroduction phase for coming off of the diet

Introduction phase: Elimination

The introduction phase is the most intense part of the diet because it eliminates the most foods. It's called the "gut healing phase" and can last from three weeks to one year, depending on your symptoms.

This phase is broken down into six stages:

- Stage 1: Consume homemade bone broth, juices from probiotic foods and ginger, and drink mint or chamomile tea with honey between meals. People who are not dairy intolerant may eat unpasteurized, homemade yogurt or kefir.

- Stage 2: Add in raw organic egg yolks, ghee and stews made with vegetables and meat or fish.

• Stage 3: All previous foods plus avocado, fermented vegetables, GAPS-recipe pancakes and scrambled eggs made with ghee, duck fat, or goose fat.

• Stage 4: Add in grilled and roasted meats, cold-pressed olive oil, vegetable juice, and GAPS-recipe bread.

• Stage 5: Introduce cooked apple purée, raw vegetables starting with lettuce and peeled cucumber, fruit juice, and small amounts of raw fruit, but no citrus.

• Stage 6: Finally, introduce more raw fruit, including citrus.

During the introduction phase, the diet requires you to introduce foods slowly, starting with small amounts and building up gradually.

The diet recommends that you move from one stage to the next once you are tolerating the foods you have introduced. You are considered to be tolerating a food when you have a normal bowel movement.

Once the introduction diet is complete, you can move to the full GAPS diet.

Maintenance phase: The full GAPS diet

The full GAPS diet can last 1.5–2 years. During this part of the diet, people are advised to base the majority of their diet on the following foods:

• Fresh meat, preferably hormone-free and grass-fed

• Animal fats, such as lard, tallow, lamb fat, duck fat, raw butter, and ghee

• Fish

• Shellfish

• Organic eggs

• Fermented foods, such as kefir, homemade yogurt and sauerkraut

• Vegetables

Followers of the diet can also eat moderate amounts of nuts and GAPS-recipe baked goods made with nut flours.

There are also a number of additional recommendations that go along with the full GAPS diet. These include:

• Do not eat meat and fruit together.

• Use organic foods whenever possible.

• Eat animal fats, coconut oil, or cold-pressed olive oil at every meal.

• Consume bone broth with every meal.

• Consume large amounts of fermented foods, if you can tolerate them.

• Avoid packaged and canned foods.

While on this phase of the diet, you should avoid all other foods, particularly refined carbs, preservatives, and artificial colorings

Reintroduction phase: Coming off GAPS

If you're following the GAPS diet to the letter, you'll be on the full diet for at least 1.5–2 years before you start reintroducing other foods.

The diet suggests that you start the reintroduction phase after you have experienced normal digestion and bowel movements for at least 6 months.

Like the other stages of this diet, the final stage can also be a long process as you reintroduce foods slowly over a number of months.

The diet suggests introducing each food individually in a small amount. If you don't note any digestive issues over 2–3 days, you may gradually increase your portions.

The diet doesn't detail the order or the exact foods you should introduce. However, it states that you should start with new potatoes and fermented, gluten-free grains.

Even once you're off the diet, you're advised to continue avoiding all highly processed and refined high-sugar foods, retaining the whole-foods principles of the protocol.

GAPS supplements

The diet's founder states that the most important aspect of the GAPS protocol is the diet.

However, the GAPS protocol also recommends various supplements. These include:

• Probiotics

• Essential fatty acids

• Digestive enzymes

• Cod liver oil

Probiotics

Probiotic supplements are added to the diet to help restore the balance of beneficial bacteria in your gut.

It's recommended that you choose a probiotic containing strains from a range of bacteria, including Lactobacilli, Bifidobacteria, and Bacillus subtilis varieties.

You're advised to look for a product that contains at least 8 billion bacterial cells per gram and to introduce the probiotic slowly into your diet.

Essential fatty acids and cod liver oil

People on the GAPS diet are advised to take daily supplements of both fish oil and cod liver oil to ensure they're getting enough.

The diet also suggests you take small amounts of a cold-pressed nut and seed oil blend that has a 2:1 ratio of omega-3 to omega-6 fatty acids.

Digestive enzymes

The diet's founder claims that people with GAPS conditions also have low stomach acid production. To remedy this, she suggests followers of the diet take a supplement of betaine HCl with added pepsin before each meal.

This supplement is a manufactured form of hydrochloric acid, one of the main acids produced in your stomach. Pepsin is an enzyme also produced in the stomach, which works to break down and digest proteins.

Some people may want to take additional digestive enzymes to support digestion.

Does the GAPS diet work?

The two key components of the GAPS dietary protocol are an elimination diet and dietary supplements.

The elimination diet

As yet, no studies have examined the effects of the GAPS dietary protocol on the symptoms and behaviors associated with autism.

Because of this, it's impossible to know how it could help people with autism and whether it's an effective treatment.

Other diets that have been tested in people with autism, like ketogenic diets and gluten-free, casein-free diets, have shown potential for helping improve some behaviors associated with autism.

But so far, studies have been small and dropout rates high, so it's still unclear how these diets may work and which people they may help.

There are also no other studies examining the effect of the GAPS diet on any of the other conditions it claims to treat.

Dietary supplements

The GAPS diet recommends probiotics to restore the balance of beneficial bacteria in the gut.

The effect of probiotics on the gut is a promising line of research.

One study found that children with autism had significantly different gut microbiota compared to neurotypical children, and probiotic supplementation was beneficial.

Other studies have found that particular strains of probiotics can improve the severity of autism symptoms.

The GAPS diet also suggests taking supplements of essential fats and digestive enzymes.

However, studies to date have not observed that taking essential fatty acid supplements has an effect on people with autism. Similarly, studies on the effects of digestive enzymes on autism have had mixed results.

Overall, it's not clear whether taking dietary supplements improves autistic behaviors or nutrition status. More high-quality studies are needed before the effects can be known

Does the GAPS diet have any risks?

The GAPS diet is a very restrictive protocol that requires you to cut out many nutritious foods for long periods of time.

It also provides little guidance on how to ensure your diet contains all the nutrients you need.

Because of this, the most obvious risk of going on this diet is malnutrition. This is especially true for children who are growing fast and need a lot of nutrients, since the diet is very restrictive.

Additionally, those with autism may already have a restrictive diet and may not readily accept new foods or changes to their diets. This could lead to extreme restriction.

Some critics have voiced the concern that consuming large amounts of bone broth could increase your intake of lead, which is toxic in high doses.

However, the risks of lead toxicity on the GAPS diet haven't been documented, so the actual risk isn't known.

Does leaky gut cause autism?

Most people who try the GAPS diet are children with autism whose parents are looking to cure or improve their child's condition.

This is because the main claims made by the diet's founder is that autism is caused by a leaky gut, and it can be cured or improved by following the GAPS diet.

Autism is a condition that results in changes to brain function that affect how the autistic person experiences the world.

Its effects can vary widely, but, in general, people with autism have difficulties with communication and social interaction.

It's a complex condition thought to result from a combination of genetic and environmental factors.

Interestingly, studies have noted that up to 70% of people with autism also have poor digestive health, which can result in symptoms including constipation, diarrhea, abdominal pain, acid reflux, and vomiting.

Untreated digestive symptoms in people with autism have also been linked with more severe behaviors, including increased irritability, tantrums, aggressive behavior, and sleep disturbances.

A small number of studies have found that some children with autism have increased intestinal permeability.

However, the results are mixed, and other studies have found no difference between intestinal permeability in children with and without autism.

There are also currently no studies that show the presence of leaky gut before the development of autism. So even if leaky gut is linked to autism in some children, it's not known if it's a cause or a symptom.

Overall, the claim that leaky gut is the cause of autism is controversial.

Some scientists think this explanation oversimplifies the causes of a complex condition. More research is needed to understand the role of leaky gut and ASD.

The bottom line

Some people feel they've benefited from the GAPS diet, though these reports are anecdotal.

However, this elimination diet is extremely restrictive for long periods of time, making it very difficult to stick to. It may be especially dangerous for the exact population it's intended for — vulnerable young people.

Many health professionals have criticized the GAPS diet because many of its claims are not supported by scientific studies.

If you're interested in trying it, seek help and support from a healthcare provider who can make sure you're meeting your nutritional needs.

A TYPICAL MENU

Start the day with a glass of still mineral or filtered water with a slice of lemon. It can be warm or cold to personal preference. If you have a juicer your patient can start the day with a glass of freshly pressed fruit/vegetable juice.

A good juice to start the day is 40% apple + 50% carrot +10% beetroot (all raw of course). You can make all sorts of juice mixes, but generally try to have 50% of therapeutic ingredients: carrot, small amount of beetroot (no more than 5% of the juice mixture), celery, cabbage, lettuce, greens (spinach, parsley, dill, basil, fresh nettle leaves, beet tops, carrot tops), white and red cabbage, and 50% of some tasty ingredients to disguise the taste of therapeutic ingredients: pineapple, apple, orange, grapefruit, grapes, mango, etc. Your patient can have these juices straight or diluted with water.

Every day our bodies go through a 24 hour cycle of activity and rest, feeding and cleaning up (detoxifying). From about 4am till about 10am the body is in the cleaning up or detoxification mode. Eating fresh fruit, drinking water and freshly pressed juices will assist in this process. Loading the body with food at that time interferes with the detoxification. That is why many of us do not feel hungry first thing in the morning. It is better to have breakfast around 10am when your body has completed the detox stage and is ready for feeding. At that stage we usually start feeling hungry. Children maybe ready for their breakfast earlier than adults.

Breakfast choices

• Eggs cooked to personal liking and served with sausages and vegetables, some cooked, some fresh as a salad (tomato, cucumber, onions, celery, any fresh salad greens, etc.) and/or avocado and/or meat. The yolks are best uncooked and the whites - cooked. Use plenty of cold pressed olive oil as a dressing on the salad and eggs. Mix a tablespoon of pre-soaked or sprouted sunflower and/or sesame and/or pumpkin seeds with the salad. Sausages (full fat) should be made of pure minced meat with only salt and pepper added. Make sure that there is no commercial seasoning or MSG (MonosodiumGlutamate) in the sausages. I recommend finding a local butcher, who would make pure meat sausages for you on order. If diarrhoea is present then the vegetables should be well cooked and the person should not have seeds at this stage.

• Avocado with meat, fish or shellfish, vegetables raw and cooked, lemon and cold pressed olive oil. Serve a cup of warm meat stock as a drink with food.

• Pancakes made with ground nuts. These pancakes are delicious with some butter and honey, or as a savoury snack. If you blend some fresh or defrosted berries with honey, it will make a delicious jam to have with pancakes. Weak tea with lemon, ginger tea or mint tea.

• Any of the home baked goods: muffins, fruit cake or bread.

Lunch

• Home-made vegetable soup or stew in a home-made meat stock.

• Avocado with meat, fish, shellfish and raw or cooked vegetables. Use olive oil with some lemon squeezed over it as a dressing. Serve a cup of warm home-made meat stock as a drink.

• Any meat/fish dish made with vegetables.

Dinner

One of the dishes from the lunch or breakfast choice.

For snacks between meals your patient can have fruit, nuts and home-baked products.

A few words about vegetarianism

I had a few families where parents are dedicated vegetarians and want their children to be vegetarians as well. These cases are the most difficult to treat because after eliminating all grains, sugar and starchy vegetables from the diet there is not much left to eat. What these parents need to know is some statistics:

1. Vegetarian children are more prone to health problems than children who eat meat, particularly to psychomotor impairment.

2. Vegetarians are prone to muscle loss and bone damage. They, on average, have lower muscle strength.

3. According to census data vegetarians die younger than people who eat meat.

From my clinical observations I have yet to meet a healthy vegetarian. In the process of evolution we humans have evolved to be omnivores, eating everything we can find in the environment: plants, eggs and meats. Our physiology is designed to work on these foods. To be healthy and full of energy we require a substantial amount of protein every day. GAPS people are particularly in need of high-quality proteins from meats, fish and eggs because their digestive systems are not in a fit state to handle hard-to- digest proteins from plants. Imposing vegetarianism on your GAPS child will undermine his or her chance of recovery.

Vegetarians have every right to follow their beliefs and to make decisions about their personal eating habits. But I strongly advise not imposing these beliefs on your GAPS child! Get your child healthy and well first through using GAPS nutritional protocol! Then allow your child grow and be mature enough to make his/her own decision whether to be a vegetarian or an omnivore. After all our children have a right to chose for themselves!

THE APPROPRIATE DIET FOR GAP SYNDROME

Recommended foods

Almonds, including almond butter and oil Apples

Apricots, fresh or dried

Artichoke, French

Asiago cheese

Asparagus

Aubergine (eggplant)

Avocados, including avocado oil

Bananas (ripe only with brown spots on the skin) Beans, dried white (navy), string beans and lima beans Beef, fresh or frozen

Beets or beetroot

Berries, all kinds

Black, white and red pepper: ground and pepper corns Black radish

Blue cheese

Bok Choy

Brazil nuts

Brick cheese

Brie cheese

Broccoli

Brussels sprouts

Butter

Cabbage
Camembert cheese
Canned fish in oil or water only Capers
Carrots
Cashew nuts, fresh only Cauliflower
Cayenne pepper
Celeriac
Celery
Cellulose in supplements
Cheddar cheese
Cherimoya (custard apple or sharifa) Cherries

Chestnuts
Chicken, fresh or frozen
Cinnamon
Citric acid
Coconut, fresh or dried (shredded) without any additives
Coconut milk
Coconut oil
Coffee, weak and freshly made, not instant
Collard greens
Colby cheese
Courgette
Coriander, fresh or dried
Cucumber
Dates, fresh or dried without any additives (not soaked in syrup) Dill, fresh or dried
Duck, fresh or frozen
Edam cheese
Eggplant (aubergine)
Eggs, fresh

Filberts
Fish, fresh or frozen, canned in its juice or oil
Game, fresh or frozen
Garlic
Ghee, home-made
Gin, occasionally
Ginger root, fresh
Goose, fresh or frozen
Gorgonzola cheese
Gouda cheese
Grapefruit
Grapes
Havarti cheese
Hazelnuts
Herbal teas
Herbs, fresh or dried without additives
Honey, natural
fuices freshly pressed from permitted fruit and vegetables
Kale
Kiwi fruit

Kumquats
Lamb, fresh or frozen
Lemons
Lentils
Lettuce, all kinds
Lima beans (dried and fresh)
Limburger cheese
Limes
Mangoes
Meats, fresh or frozen

Melons

Monterey (lack) cheese

Muenster cheese

Mushrooms

Mustard seeds, pure powder and gourmet types without any non-allowed ingredients

Nectarines

Nut flour or ground nuts (usually ground blanched almonds)

Nutmeg

Nuts, all kinds freshly shelled, not roasted, salted or coated

Olive oil, virgin cold-pressed

Olives preserved without sugar or any other non-allowed ingredients Onions

Oranges

Papayas

Parmesan cheese

Parsley

Peaches

Peanut butter, without additives

Peanuts, fresh or roasted in their shells

Pears

Peas, dried split and fresh green

Pecans

Peppers (green, yellow, red and orange)

Pheasant, fresh or frozen

Pickles, without sugar or any other non-allowed ingredients

Pigeon, fresh or frozen

Pineapples, fresh Pork, fresh or frozen

Port du Salut cheese

Poultry, fresh or frozen

Prunes, dried without any additives or in their own juice
Pumpkin
Quail, fresh or frozen
Raisins
Rhubarb
Roquefort cheese
Romano cheese
Satsumas
Scotch, occasionally
Shellfish, fresh or frozen
Spices, single and pure without any additives
Spinach
Squash (summer and winter)
Stilton cheese
String beans
Swiss cheese
Tangerines
Tea, weak freshly made, not instant
Tomato puree, pure without any additives apart from salt
Tomato juice, without any additives apart from salt
Tomatoes
Turkey, fresh or frozen
TUrnips
Ugly fruit
Uncreamed cottage cheese (dry curd)
Vinegar (cider or white); make sure there is no allergy Vodka, very occasionally
Walnuts
Watercress
Wine dry: red or white
Yoghurt, home-made

Zucchini

Foods to avoid

Acesulphame Acidophilus milk Agar-agar
Agave syrup Algae
Aloe Vera
Amaranth
Apple juice
Arrowroot
Aspartame
Astragalus
Baked beans
Baker's yeast
Baking power and raising agents of all kind Balsamic vinegar
Barley
Bean flour and sprouts
Bee pollen
Beer
Bhindior okra
Bicarbonate of soda
Bitter Gourd
Black eye beans
Bologna
Bouillon cubes or granules
Brandy
Buckwheat
Bulgur
Burdock root
Butter beans
Buttermilk
Canellini beans

Canned vegetables and fruit

Carob

Carrageenan

Cellulose gum

Cereals, including all breakfast cereals

Cheeses, processed and cheese spreads Chestnut flour

Chevre cheese

Chewing gum

Chickpeas

Chickoryroot

Chocolate

Cocoa powder

Coffee, instant and coffee substitutes Cooking oils

Cordials

Corn Cornstarch Corn syrup Cottage cheese Cottonseed Cous-cous Cream

Cream ofTartar Cream cheese Dextrose Drinks, soft Faba beans Feta cheese

Fish, preserved, smoked, salted, breaded and canned with sauces Flour, made out of grains

FOS (fructooligosaccharides)

Fructose

Fruit, canned or preserved Garbanzo beans

Gjetost cheese

Grains, all

Gruyere cheese

Ham

Hot dogs

Ice-cream, commercial Jams

Jellies

Jerusalem artichoke

Ketchup, commercially available
Lactose
Liqueurs
Margarines and butter replacements
Meats, processed, preserved, smoked and salted Millet
Milk from any animal, soy, rice, canned coconut milk Milk, dried
Molasses
Mozzarella cheese
Mungbeans
Neufchatel cheese
Nutra-sweet (aspartame)
Nuts, salted, roasted and coated Oats
Okra
Parsnips
Pasta, of any kind
Pectin
Postum
Potato white
Potato sweet Primost cheese Quinoa
Rice
Ricotta cheese Rye
Saccharin Sago
Sausages, commercially available Seaweed
Semolina
Sherry
Soda soft drinks
Sour cream commercial
Soy

Spelt
Starch
Sugar or sucrose of any kind
Tapioca
Tea, instant
Triticale
Turkey loaf
Vegetables, canned or preserved Wheat
Wheat germ
Whey, powder or liquid
Yams
Yoghurt, commercial

RECIPES

Condiments

Most fresh salads can be dressed with olive oil and fresh lemon juice. When home-made yoghurt is well tolerated it can also be used as a salad dressing.

Ketchup

2 cups tomato juice

2-3 tablespoons white vinegar honey to taste bay leaf (optional) salt and pepper to taste. Mix all the ingredients except the honey and simmer on the stove until thick, stirring often to prevent sticking. When almost the desired thickness, add honey to taste and complete cooking. Ladle into sterilised jars and seal immediately or place in small containers and freeze.

Guacamole

2 ripe avocados juice ofi orange

1 clove of crushed garlic, small amount of water

In the food processor blend together all the ingredients. Reduce the amount of garlic, if the guacamole is too hot. Use as a dip for vegetables and a spread for home-made bread.

Mayonnaise

1 whole egg

1 cup olive oil or slightly more

1 tablespoon white vinegar or fresh lemon juice IU teaspoon dry mustard powder, salt and pepper to taste a little honey to taste.

Blend in your food processor for a few seconds: egg, lemon juice (or vinegar), mustard, salt, pepper and honey. While the machine is running, (Recipe courtesy of Elaine Gottschall) add the oil in a fine stream. Do not add oil quickly; it should take at least 60 seconds. As mayonnaise thickens, the sound of the machine will deepen. Suggestions:

Use to thicken gravy: add 2 tablespoons of mayonnaise to about 1 cup of meat stock and heat gently for about 1-2 minutes, stirring constantly.

Use as a base for tartar sauce by adding lk cup chopped dill pickles (unsweetened) and I U cup of chopped onion.

Use as mock Hollandaise sauce by adding grated cheddar cheese (if well tolerated). Spread over vegetables such as cooked cauliflower or broccoli. Cover and heat in oven.

Mix with home-made yoghurt (1 part mayonnaise, 1 part yoghurt) and use as salad dressing.

Salsa

4 medium-size tomatoes half a pepper (green, red, orange or yellow) 1 medium onion (white or red)

1-3 cloves of garlic dill and parsley

olive oil

salt and pepper to taste

Put all ingredients into the food processor and chop coarsely. Can be served with meats and vegetables. You can also use it for cookingmeats. To do that bring salsa to simmer, add diced meat (beef, pork, lamb or chicken) and 3-4 tablespoons of butter (or goose/duckfat), cover and simmer for 30 minutes.

Aubergine dip

2 aubergines (eggplants) salt

3 medium-size tomatoes 3-4 cloves of garlic

7 cup olive oil fresh dill or parsley

Cut the aubergines into 1 cm-thick slices, rub well with salt and duck fat. Place on a baking tray and bake at i5OO C for 30-40 minutes or until soft. Cool down.

In the food processor blend together the baked aubergines, tomatoes, garlic, herbs and olive oil. Serve with meats and fish and as a dip with vegetables.

Basic liver pate wog liver

1 largeonion finely chopped

3 cloves of garlic finely chopped

Fry the liver, onion and garlic in ghee (butter, goose or duck fat) until well cooked through. Blend in a food processor with mayonnaise.

To make variations you can add one of the following when blending:

• 1 raw tomato

• 4-5 cooked prunes (unsweetened and without stones)

• Raw garlic

• Greens (dill, parsley, basil) • raw onion

• Peeled, cored and grated apple

2. Salads

Salads should be served when diarrhoea is no longer present.

To increase the nutritional value of your salads it is good to sprinkle coarsely chopped walnuts or seeds on top. Seeds: sunflower seeds, pump- kin and sesame should be soaked in water over night. It makes them more nourishing and easier to digest.

Beetroot salad

8 small beetroots

1 cup of shelled walnuts 2cloves of garlic

8 dried prunes without stones mayonnaise

7» teaspoon of salt

Wash the beetroots and cut all tops and ends off. Cook the beetroot by steaming until a knife goes through easily. Alternatively you can buy* already cooked beetroots (in water, not in vinegar!). Grate the beetroot through a coarse grater. In the food processor chop together the walnuts, garlic and prunes. Mix well with the grated beetroot. Add salt, mayonnaise and mix. Enjoy with meats and vegetables.

Tuna salad

200g canned tuna in its own juice or water 1 large onion

2 large carrots

2 hard-boiled eggs

mayonnaise

Drain the tuna and mash with a fork. Chop the onion finely. Cook the car- rots. Peel and chop the hard-boiled eggs.

On a flat dish put a layer of tuna (use half the tuna) and top it up with half of the chopped onion. Cover with mayonnaise. Grate one carrot on top and cover with mayonnaise. Make a layer of one chopped hard-boiled egg and cover with mayonnaise. Repeat with the same layers of tuna, onion, carrot and egg. Decorate on the top with some dill or parsley. Make sure that every layer is well covered with mayonnaise.

Salad with cabbage and apple

loog of white cabbage

1 large apple

a cup of home-made yoghurt or cremefraiche 1 teaspoon of honey

a pinch of salt

2 table-spoons of raisins

Grate the cabbage. Peel, core and grate the apple. Slightly fry the raisins in butter to make them soft. Mix honey and salt with yoghurt. Mix all ingredi- ents together.

Salad with tomatoes and cucumber

2 tomatoes or a long cucumber, 1 stick of celery spring onion dill or parsley salt.

Cut cucumbers into IU cm thick slices. Cut tomato into mouth-size pieces and slice the celery into small pieces. Sprinkle with salt. Chop the spring onions, dill and parsley. Mix all ingredients and dress with cold pressed olive oil.

Russian salad

1 long cucumber

1 large carrot cooked (steamed)

loog cooked meat or sausages (leftovers are good) 1 onion

2 hard-boiled eggs

2 tablespoons of sauerkraut (optional) fresh dill and/or parsley

'Is teaspoon salt

mayonnaise

yoghurt or cr&mefraiche

Cut cucumber and carrot into small cubes. Cut the meat and/or sausages into small cubes. Finely chop the onion. Peel and cut the eggs into small cubes. Finely chop dill and parsley. In a separate pot mix mayonnaise and yoghurt in equal proportions and add salt Mix all ingredients together.

Carrot salad

1 large carrot

1 tablespoon of raisins

1 tablespoon of coarsely chopped walnuts yoghurt

Slightly fry the raisins in butter to make them soft. Finely grate the carrot. Mix the carrot, raisins, walnuts and yoghurt.

3. Soups

I strongly recommend to making your soups based on a home-made meat / stock. Meat stock aids digestion and has been known for centuries as a healing folk remedy for the digestive tract. Also home-made meat stock is extremely nourishing, it is full of minerals, vitamins, amino-acids and various other nutrients in a very bio-available form. Do not use commercially available soup stock granules or bouillon cubes, they are highly processed and are full of detrimental ingredients.

Once you have made your meat stock, it can be frozen or it will keep well in a refrigerator for at least a week. You can make soups, gravies and stews with this meat stock or warm up a cup of it to give your GAPS patient as a drink with meals or between meals. If you make sure that you always have some meat stock in your fridge, you will find that it is very easy and quick to make nourishing meals for your GAPS child or adult and the rest of the family.

You need meat and bones to make a good meat stock. Beef, lamb, pork, game, poultry and fish are all highly suitable and will make stocks with different flavours and different nutritional compositions. So, make sure that you alternate between different meats to provide a whole spectrum of nourishment. Bones and joints are particularly important as they enrich the stock with the kind of nourishing substances which meat alone cannot provide. In fact it can be very inexpensive to make a good quality meat stock as you use the parts of the animal which butchers usually give away almost free. The meat and bones can be fresh or frozen and there is no need to defrost them prior to cooking. Apart from bones and meat all you need is a large pot full of water and a bit of salt and pepper.

How to make a meat stock

Lamb, pork, beef or game

Put the joints, bones and meat into a large pot, add 5-10 pepper corns, add salt to taste and fill it up with water. Heat up to a boiling point. Cover the pan, reduce the heat to a minimum and simmer for 3 hours at least. The longer you cook the meat and bones, the more they will "give out" to the stock and the more nourishing the stock will be. Take the bones and meat out and pour the stock through a sieve into a separate pan to remove any small bones and pepper corns.

Chicken stock

Put a whole or half a chicken into a large pot, fill it up with water, add salt and heat it up to boiling point. Simmer for 1V2-2 hours. Take the chicken out and put the stock through a sieve. Keep in the refrigerator. The chicken, cooked this way is delicious and can be served for dinner with vegetables and a hot cup of your freshly made chicken stock.

Fish stock

To make a good fish stock you need bones, fins, skins and heads of the fish, not the meat. So buy your fish whole, cut the meat off to cook as a separate meal and use the rest of the fish to make your fish stock. Your fishmonger can do all the trimming for you. Put the heads, bones, fins and skin of the fish into a large pan, add 8-10 pepper corns and fill the pan with water. Bring up to boil, reduce the heat to a minimum and simmer for i-i72 hours. Add salt to taste at the end of cooking. Take the fish out and sieve the stock. Take the meat off the fish skeleton to use for soup making.

The basic soup recipe

To make a soup bring some of your home-made meat stock to the boil, add chopped or sliced vegetables and simmer for another 20-25 minutes. You can choose any combination of available vegetables: onion, cabbage, carrot, broccoli, cauliflower, pumpkin, courgettes, marrow, squash, leeks, etc. If you are planning to blend your soup, then you can cut vegetables roughly into any size pieces. If you prefer to have your soup without blend- ing, then make sure that you cut or dice your vegetables into nice small pieces before cooking. If your meat stock was made with lamb, pork or beef you can add a handful of dried French or Italian mushrooms for a wonderful flavour. It is customary to crush the dried mushrooms by hand before adding to the soup. At the end of cooking add 1-2 table spoon- fuls of chopped garlic, bring to the boil and turn the heat off. Blend with a soup blender until smooth unless you planned to have it without blending.

You can serve your soup with any combination of the following:

• Some chopped parsley, coriander or dill

• Hard-boiled egg cut into pieces

• A spoonful of your home-made goat's yoghurt or creme fraiche

• Cooked meat cut into small pieces

• Red onion cut into very small pieces

• Spring onion cut into small pieces

• A spoonful of cooked and ground liver

From this basic recipe you can improvise and develop your own recipes. Here I will just provide a few ideas.

A spring nettle soup

I'L l of home-made meat stock

Large bunch of spring nettles

2 tablespoons of dried French of Italian mushrooms 1 medium onion

1 medium carrot

2 courgettes or 7, of a marrow or squash

4 eggs, hard boiled

Young shoots of stinging nettles appearing in spring are full of wonderful nourishment. They are high in iron, magnesium, copper, zinc, vitamin C, carotenoids and other useful substances. For this recipe collect a large bunch of spring nettles. You will have to wear gloves and a long-sleeved shirt to do this. Rinse the nettles and shake the excess water off. Using scissors cut the leaves and tender shoots of the nettles into small pieces discarding the hard stems. Reserve for the recipe.

Cut the marrow, squash or courgettes into small cubes, thinly slice the carrot and chop the onion. Bring the home-made meat stock to a boil. Add all the vegetables and the French or Italian dried mushrooms, crumbling them with your hands before adding to the meat stock. Simmer under a tight lid for 15-20 minutes. Add your prepared nettles, mix and immediately take off the heat. Serve with 1-2 tablespoons of hard-boiled egg cut into small pieces and a spoonful of home-made yoghurt (if well tolerated).

Russian Borsch

tit I of home-made meat stock

1 medium onion finely chopped

1medium carrot finely sliced

'U ofmedium-size white cabbage finely sliced

2 medium-size beetroots or4 small beetroots raw or cooked

3 cloves of garlic

1 finely chopped tomato

If the beetroot is cooked (in water, not in vinegar):

Bring the meat stock to boil and add the onion, carrot and cabbage. Cover and simmer for 20 minutes. In the meantime slice the cooked beetroots into long thin strips. Add into the soup, mix well and simmer for another 5 minutes. Take off the heat. Crush the 3 cloves of garlic and add to the soup together with the chopped tomato. Serve with a large spoon of creme fraiche or home-made yoghurt (if well tolerated) and some chopped parsley and/or a thick slice of hard-boiled egg.

If the beetroot is raw:

Wash and peel the beetroot. Slice into long thin strips by hand or using your food processor. Bring the meat stock to boil and add the beetroot. Simmer for 10-15 minutes, then add the rest of the vegetables (onion, carrot and cabbage). Simmer for further 20 minutes or until the cabbage is cooked. Take off the heat. Crush the 3 cloves of garlic and add to the soup together with the chopped tomato. Serve with a large spoon of creme fraiche or home made yoghurt (if well tolerated), some chopped parsley and/or a thick slice of hard-boiled egg.

Fish soup

1l of home-made fish stock

1 large onion finely chopped

1 carrot thinly sliced

1 courgette or an equivalent amount of marrow or squash, cut into small cubes

Bring the fish stock to boil and add the onion, carrot and squash, marrow or courgettes. Simmer under a lid for 10-15 minutes and take off the heat. Add the cooked fish meat which you took off the bones when you made the fish stock. Serve with a spoonful of home-made yoghurt (if well tolerated) and/or with a hard-boiled egg (sliced or chopped).

If there is no meat left on the bones you can use the meat (skinless and boneless) of any available fish. Cut the meat into small cubes and add into the boiling fish stock at the same time as vegetables.

Meatball soup

400 g of minced meat (mixture of pork and beef is best) 1 large onion finely chopped

1 large carrot thinly sliced

1 cup winter squash or courgette cut into small cubes 1cup of finely chopped cabbage (optional)

2 tablespoons of chopped garlic

In a pan bring 2 litres of water up to boil. Add salt and cayenne pepper to taste.

With your hands shape meatballs about 2 cm in diameter and add them, one at a time, into the boiling water. Cover and simmer on low heat for 30 minutes. Add all the vegetables apart from garlic, cover and simmer for another 20 minutes. Add the garlic and switch the heat off. Let it sit for 5-10 minutes then add 2-3 tablespoons of sauerkraut. Serve with a spoonful of home-made yoghurt and finely chopped dill.

Lite beautiful winter squash soup

TIL I of home-made meat stock (turkey or chicken stock work best for this recipe)

1 leak, washed and sliced

Broccoli, 3-4 medium sized rosettes

1 medium-size carrot, sliced

Va of a medium size buttercup squash ora'h of butternut squash or any winter squash with sweet orange flesh

3 garlic cloves peeled

Peel and de-seed the squash, cut it into chunks. Wash and cut into pieces all the vegetables. Put them into your soup pan, add the meat stock and bring to boil. Reduce the heat to a minimum, cover with the lid and simmer for about 30 minutes. Blend with a soup blender. If your family is at the stage of tolerating home-made goat's yoghurt, then add lh a cup into the soup. Serve warm. It is particularly soothing if the child has a tummy ache or diarrhoea.

Meat jelly

pig trotters (2-4) 1 large carrot garlic

salt and black peppercorns

Put pig trotters into a large pan, fill it up with water, add salt and a tea- spoon of black peppercorns. Bring up to boil, reduce heat to a minimum, cover with a lid and let it simmer for 3 hours.

In the meantime cook a large carrot by steaming, cool it down and cut into thin slices. You can cut it into decorative slices if you have the tools for doing that.

When the meat stock is ready take the pig trotters out and pour the stock through a sieve into a separate pan. Let the trotters cool down completely. Take all the meats (including the skin and other soft tissues) from the pig trotters, completely stripping the bones. Cut the meat into small pieces.

In a large deep tray lay the pieces of meat, the carrot pieces and thin slices of garlic. You can add more or less garlic to your family's taste. Pour the meat stock to fill the tray to 3L Place it in the refrigerator for the jelly to set. You can also set this jelly in different jelly shapes and dishes as individual servings.

This dish is wonderful to have on a hot summer's day. It contains a lot of nourishing substances, including gelatine, glucosamine, glycoproteins, phospholipids and others and is considered to be a folk remedy for digestive problems.

4 Fats for cooking

Cooking (roasting, frying, etc.) should be done with fully saturated fats, because these fats do not alter their chemical structure when heated. These fats are: pork dripping, goose fat, duck fat, natural lard, lamb fat, coconut oil, butter and ghee. You can purchase many of these fats in shops. It is also easy to make many of these fats at home which has an advantage: you know exactly what is in it. For more information on this subject please look in the chapter: Fats: the good and the bad.

Ghee

Ghee is a clarified butter. It is traditionally used in many cultures around the world for cooking and baking. Butter can be used for cooking very effectively. However, small amounts of whey in the butter often burn. Also whey contains lactose and some milk proteins, which many GAPS patients have to avoid in the initial stages of the diet. Ghee on the other hand does not contain any whey, milk protein or lactose at all, just milk fat, and does not burn.

Preheat your oven to around 6o-i20°C (250°F). Put a large block of organic, preferably unsalted butter into a metal dish or pan. Leave it in the oven for 45-60 minutes. Take it out and carefully pore the golden fat from the top (ghee), making sure that the white liquid at the bottom stays in the pan. Discard the white liquid. Keep in glass jars and refrigerate.

Goose or duck fat

Roast a goose or a duck in the oven in the usual way. Take the bird out and pour the fat through a cheese-cloth or a fine metal sieve. Keep in glass jars and refrigerate. Use for cooking meats and vegetables. These fats give a nice flavour to roasted vegetables in particular.

Pork, lamb or beef fat (lard)

You can collect these fats in much the same way as the duck and goose fats. You need any bits of fat from the animal. It is particularly good to use internal fat layer from the animal, which the butcher often gives away almost free. You will be amazed how much cooking fat you will collect from a fairly small piece. It is wise to use organic animals for this purpose, as fat is a natural body storage for various toxins. Investing in a small piece of organic fat once or twice a year will not cost you much and will last for many months.

Roast the fat on a fairly low heat (i2o-i30°C) for 2-3 hours depending on the size of the piece. Pour the fat through the cheese-cloth or a fine metal sieve. Store in glass jars and refrigerate.

Coconut oil is very good for cooking. It contains largely saturated fats and hence does not change its chemical structure, when heated. However, make sure that you buy good quality natural coconut oil, as a lot of brands, sold in the west have been hydrogenated to increase shelf-life.

5. Main dishes

An Italian meat casserole

This is an alternative way of making an excellent meat stock as well as preparing a meal for the whole family. You can use any of the following: a leg or a shoulder of lamb, a joint of pork, a joint of beef, a pheasant, 2-4 pigeons, 2 quails, a joint of venison, a whole chicken, turkey legs. You need a large casserole with a lid for this dish. Put your meat joint or a whole bird(s) into the casserole, add water to fill % of the casserole, add some salt, pepper corns, dried herbs to taste, bay leaves and a sprig of rosemary. Cover with the lid and put into the oven for 5-6 hours on low heat (125-140°C or 250°F). Add various vegetables 40-50 minutes before your dinner time into the casserole: rosettes of broccoli and cauliflower, whole peeled small red or white onions, Brussels sprouts and large pieces of carrots. When ready take the meat and vegetables out and serve to your family. Put the meat stock through a sieve and serve it in bouillon cups with the dinner. Meat stock left from this dinner will keep well in the refrigerator and can be used for making soups or warming up as a nourishing drink.

Stuffed peppers

6 large peppers (a combination of green, red, yellow and orange) 7* kg ofminced meat (a mixture ofL pork andlL beefis best)

2 medium-size carrots

I large onion

salt and pepper

Grind the carrots and chop the onion. Mix them well together with the minced meat adding salt and pepper to taste.

Cut off the tops of the peppers and take out the seeds. Fill the peppers with the mixture of the meat and vegetables. Place the stuffed peppers upright into a pan. You will need the correct size pan to fit all the peppers, so they stand upright and support each other. Add 3-4 cups of water to the bottom of the pan and cover it with the lid. Bring up to boil, reduce the heat to a minimum and simmer for an hour. Serve a pepper per person with a ladle of the stock from the bottom (best to serve in a soup bowl}. Put a tablespoon of your home-made yoghurt (if well tolerated) with a clove of crushed garlic mixed into it. Garnish with chopped parsley.

Meatballs

500g of minced meat (a mixture of pork and beef is best) 1 large onion lh red pepper

1 courgette

2 tablespoons of chopped fresh garlic 1 tablespoon tomato puree

salt, pepper, 2-3 bay leaves

To make the sauce cover the bottom of the pan with water 3-4 cm high. Mix into the water tomato paste, salt and pepper. Bring to boil. With your hands shape balls out of the mincemeat about 4 cm in diameter. Put the balls one at a time into the boiling sauce. Make sure that you use a large enough pan to fit all the balls in one layer. Cover with the lid and simmer on low heat for 30 minutes.

In the meantime prepare the vegetables. Finely chop the onion and red pepper. Cut the courgette into small cubes. Chop the garlic.

After cooking the meatballs for 30 minutes add the chopped onion, pepper and courgette, mix with the sauce gently in order to preserve the shape of the meatballs. Cover and cook for another 25 minutes. Add the bay leaves and garlic. Cover and turn the heat off. Let it sit for 10 minutes before serving. Sprinkle with finely chopped coriander and serve with cooked vegetables.

Meat cutlets

5oog of minced pork

5oog of minced beef or lamb 1 large onion, finely chopped salt and pepper.

Mix all the ingredients well and make oval shaped cutlets. In a frying pan warm up some pork dripping (goose or duck fat) and fry the cutlets slightly on both sides. Place the cutlets into a greased baking tray add 72 a cup of water and bake in the oven for 40 minutes at 150-170*0 (300-350o F). Serve with cooked vegetables and a salad.

Fish cutlets

2-3 fairly large freshwater or sea fish, a mixture of different fish works very well

3-5 tablespoons of butter (ghee, goose fat, duck fat, pork dripping or coconut oil)

1-2 cups of shredded coconut

salt and pepper

Cut all the meat off the fish, remove skin and large bones. Use the bones, heads and skin for making a very nourishing fish stock (recipe in the soup section). Alternatively you can buy fish fillets already without skin and large bones.

In the food processor put the meat of the fish, one egg, butter, salt and pepper to your taste and grind it to make mince. If you have a meat mincer it will do the same job for you. With your hands make oval-shaped flat cut- lets about 2 cm thick, roll them in shredded coconut and slightly fry them on both sides. Use coconut oil (or butter, ghee, pork dripping, lard, goose fat or duck fat) for frying. Move the cutlets into a large oven tray, greased with any of the mentioned fats. Add half a cup of water and put into pre- heated oven. Bake for 20-30 minutes at iso°C (300T).

Swedish Gravlax - the best way to eat fresh salmon skinless and boneless salmon fillet 11 water at room temperature

th tablespoons of salt

1 tablespoon of honey

fresh dill and coarsely ground black pepper

The fish has to be very fresh. Cut the fish into 0.5cm thick slices and place in a dip tray (any baking tray will do). Sprinkle with finely chopped dill and black pepper. Dissolve the salt and the honey in the water to make a brine. Cover the fish with the brine and leave at room temperature for I-i'A hours. Pour the water out and serve the fish with some lettuce and mayonnaise.

This dish works particularly well with wild salmon. Because the fish is not cooked all the essential fatty acids and other nutrients are preserved. Refrigerate and consume within two days.

Baked beans or French Cassoulet

soog white (navy) beans

1 duck

1 tablespoon cider vinegar

1 teaspoon sea salt

2 tablespoons tomato puree

cayenne pepper and black pepper

5-6 bay leaves, a sprig ofrosemary, a teaspoon ofthyme

Soak the beans in water for 12-24 hours, drain, rinse well in cold water and drain again.

Cut all the meat from the duck: the legs, wings, breasts and all the fat. Cut the meat into chunks and the fat into small pieces. The carcass of the duck and the giblets you can use for making meat stock later.

In a large pan put 2 litres of water, cider vinegar, sea salt, tomato puree, a pinch of each cayenne pepper and black pepper, bay leaves, rosemary and thyme. Mix in the beans and the duck pieces (the meat and the fat). Cover the pan with a lid and put it into an oven. Cook at i2o°C (25o°F) for 4-5 hours. Check occasionally. If the beans are getting dry, add more water.

Serve hot. The baked beans left from this meal will keep in the fridge for a long time and can be served with other dishes.

Casserole with turkey legs

2 turkey legs

11 of water

l heaped tablespoon 1 teaspoon of salt

6-io pepper corns

of tomato

puree

a pinch of cayenne

fresh or dried herbs: oregano, rosemary, bay leaves

a combination of available vegetables: choose from carrots, winter squash, pumpkin, courgette, marrow, peeled small/medium onions, cauliflower, broccoli, peppers, aubergine and Brussels sprouts

In a large oval casserole put the water, salt, tomato puree, pepper corns, cayenne pepper and herbs. Mix well. Put the turkey legs in. Brush the parts of the turkey legs, which are not covered with the water, with some goose fat (or duck fat, ghee, pork dripping or lard). Do not cover the casserole with the lid, leave it open. Cook in the oven at i5o°C (3oo°F) for 2-2*4 hours. About 5ominutes before the end of cooking add available vegetables, cut into large chunks. Mix them well into the sauce and leave cooking. When the vegetables are cooked so a sharp knife goes through them easily, take the casserole out. Serve the meat and the vegetables with some freshly chopped parsley and garlic.

Liver pudding

loog liver (calf or lamb)

2 tablespoons of butter (or ghee, l medium-size onion

salt

parsley

goose/duck fat)

pepper

Soak the liver in water with some lemon juice or home-made yoghurt for a few hours to remove any bitter taste. You can also soak the liver in the liquid left from draining your home-made yoghurt. Wash the liver, dry with a paper towel and blend in the food processor into a pulp. Put through a sieve to remove any hard bits. Add salt, egg yolk, butter, finely chopped parsley and finely chopped onion. Whip the egg white stiff and fold into the mixture. Put the mixture into a suitable dish, cover with a sheet of baking paper and cook with steam. You can use a steamer or a large pan. To steam in a pan put some water at the bottom of the pan and place the dish in it. Make sure that you don't have too much water in the pan, so it does not get into the dish with the liver. Cover the pan with a lid and put it on the stove. Steam for about one hour. Serve with cooked vegetables or vegetable risotto.

Liver in a clay pot

loog liver (calf or lamb)

loog lamb's hearts

1 large onion

10 dried prunes with stones

1 large pot of natural yoghurt or soured cream (you can useyourhome- madeyoghurt or replace with lh cup ofbutterlghee)

a pinch ofallspice, salt, pepper

Soak the liver in water with some lemon juice or home-made yoghurt for a few hours to remove any bitter taste. You can also soak the liver in the liquid left from draining your home-made yoghurt. Wash, dry and cut into small pieces using scissors. Cut lamb's hearts into small pieces using scissors. In a suitable size clay pot put the liver and lamb's heats, finely chopped onion and prunes. Into the yoghurt add salt, pepper, allspice and mix well. Add into the clay pot and mix with the meats. Cover the pot with the lid or foil. Bake in the oven for about l hour at i6o°C (320°F),

Quick liver recipe

loog liver

I large onion

6-7 cloves of garlic

'/2 cup ofbu tterlghee (use goose/duck fat if avoidingbutter)

fresh parsley or dill

Soak the liver in water with some lemon juice or home-made yoghurt for a few hours to remove any bitter taste. You can also soak the liver in the liquid left from draining your home-made yoghurt. Wash and dry the liver and cut into small pieces using scissors. In a frying pan melt the butter/ghee, add the sliced onion and finely chopped garlic. Fry slightly until the onion and garlic start turning golden. Add the liver, salt, pepper and stir-fry for about 4-5 minutes. Sprinkle chopped parsley or dill on top and drizzle with olive oil. Serve immediately.

6. Vegetables

Cooked vegetables are nourishing, warming and easy to digest, they are gentle on the gut lining and should be a regular part of the diet. You can cook your vegetables by steaming, stir-frying, stewing, roasting, grilling or as a soup. Instead of boiling vegetables I recommend steaming them as boiling removes a lot of nutrients into the water which then gets thrown away. The best vegetables to steam are broccoli, cauliflower, Brussels sprouts, fresh green beans (runner beans, string beans, etc.) carrots, asparagus, French artichokes and beetroot.

If diarrhoea is not present raw vegetables should also be a normal part of every meal, they would provide a lot of active enzymes, which will help you to digest your food. Carrots, cucumber, tomato, greens, cabbage, onion, garlic, lettuce, baby spinach, celery, cauliflower can all be served as salads or cut into rosettes and sticks to eat with a dip (mayonnaise, guacamole, liver pate, aubergine dip, etc).

Sauerkraut

Sauerkraut is a fermented white and/or red cabbage, commonly con- sumed in Germany, Russia and Eastern Europe. It is a wonderful healing remedy for the digestive tract full of digestive enzymes, probiotic bacteria, vitamins and minerals. Eating it with meats will improve digestion as it has a strong ability to stimulate stomach acid production. For people with low stomach acidity I recommend having a few tablespoons of sauerkraut (or juice from it) 10-15 minutes before meals. For children, initially add 1-3 tablespoons of the juice from the sauerkraut into their meals.

Slice thinly a medium-size white cabbage and add two shredded carrots. You can use red cabbage or a mixture of white and red. Add salt to taste. Knead the mixture well with your hands until a lot of juice comes out. Pack this mixture into a suitable glass or stainless steel bowl, press it firmly so there is no air trapped and the cabbage is drowned in its own juice. Place a plate on top of the cabbage, which is about lcm smaller in diameter than the bowl. The gap will allow the fermentation gases to escape. On top of the plate place something heavy enough to keep the cabbage constantly submerged in its juice. Cover the whole thing with a kitchen towel to keep it in the dark. It should take 5-7 days inside the house for the sauerkraut to be ready, (it will take two weeks in a cool place, like a garage). Sauerkraut is delicious with any meal and it can be added to your homemade soups and stews.

A nice way to cook cabbage

V2 a cabbage finely sliced

1 large carrot finely sliced

1k onion finely chopped

1 tomato finely chopped

1 tablespoon of chopped garlic salt and pepper to taste

Cover the bottom of the pan with home-made meat stock and bring to the boil. Add cabbage, carrot, onion, salt and pepper. Cover and cook on a low heat for 30 minutes. Add the chopped tomato and garlic, mix, cook for another 3 minutes and take off the heat. Mix in lk cup of homemade yoghurt or soured cream. Serve with meat.

Quick vegetable risotto

2 courgettes or a quarter of a medium-size marrow

1 large onion

10 cloves of garlic

1 pepper red, yellow or green (or a combination of different coloured peppers)

1 tablespoon of tomato puree salt and pepper

In a frying pan melt about 50g of butter. Mix in sliced courgettes or marrow, onion, garlic, sliced peppers, tomato puree, season to taste with salt and pepper. Cover with a lid and leave for 10 minutes on minimum heat. Alternatively you can stir-fry it on a low heat. Mix well and serve with plenty of cold pressed virgin olive oil and freshly chopped dill or parsley. Enjoy with meat and fish.

Cauliflower "potatoes"

1 large cauliflower cut into pieces

V< cup butter or ll, cup home-made yoghurt salt, pepper to taste parsley and paprika garnish

Cook cauliflower until just tender. Drain.

Puree in blender or food processor. Add butter or yoghurt, salt and pepper and blend thoroughly. Reheat and serve. Garnish with parsley and paprika. The pureed cauliflower may be placed in a baking dish, sprinkled with grated cheddar cheese and heated in the oven until the cheese melts.

Baked vegetables

You can bake any combination of the following vegetables: onions, white or red or shallots peppers, red, yellow, orange or green Brussels sprouts courgettes or marrow pumpkin winter squashes large mushrooms turnips aubergines (eggplant).

Peal the onion and cut into halves or quarters. Shallots do not need to be peeled, just bake them in their skins.

Cut the peppers into quarters, remove seeds.

Peel the outer leaves from Brussels sprouts.

Peel and cut into large chunks courgettes, marrow and pumpkin.

Remove the seeds from the pumpkin and the marrow. Rub courgettes and marrow with salt.

Peel and slice winter squash, remove the seeds.

Peel the turnips and cut like potato chips.

Cut the aubergine into chunks and rub with salt.

Rub plenty of goose or duck fat on the vegetables, place them in a baking tray and bake at 150°C (300°F) for 20-40 minutes or until a sharp knife goes through easily. Serve with meat or fish.

7. Baking at home

The basic bread I cake I muffin recipe

2% cups of ground almonds

1/4 cup of softened butter (or coconut oil, goose fat, duck fat or home-made yoghurt or cr^me fraiche) 3 eggs

Ground almonds you can buy in most health food shops. Instead of ground almonds you can use walnuts, pecans and hazelnuts, which you can grind in your food processor to a flour consistency.

Mix all the ingredients well. You may want to add more or less ground almonds to reach porridge-like consistency. Grease your baking pan with butter or ghee, line it with greased baking paper and put the mixture into it. Bake in the oven at 150°C (300°F) for about an hour. Check occasionally with a dry clean knife, if the knife comes out dry then the bread is ready.

To make variations of this bread you can add some salt, pepper, dried herbs, tomato puree, grated cheddar cheese (if well tolerated), nuts, seeds, dried fruit, fresh or frozen berries, chunks of cooking apple, grated carrot, chunks of pumpkin (without the skin and seeds). If you want to sweeten the mixtureadd Vz cup of honey into it and/or i7» cups of dried fruit (dates, apricots, raisins, figs) and/or 2 ripe bananas. If the dried fruit is too hard, soak it in water for a few hours to soften.

Improvise, try to make your own variations. You can bake this mixture as a bread or cake or in small paper cups as muffins or make a pizza base. It really is very easy and manageable even for the most inexperienced cooks.

Pizza

Make a pastry following the previous recipe. Spread it on a baking tray cov- ered with greased baking paper in a layer about 2 cm thick. Bake in the oven at i50°C (3oo°F) for about 30 minutes. Check with a dry knife if it is ready

Cool down. Spread tomato puree on the top and sprinkle with salt.

On top of the tomato puree you can put your choice of filling: slices of red/yellow/green pepper, mushrooms, pieces of cooked meat or sausages, slices of tomato, chopped greens, anchovies, fish, prawns and pineapple, etc.

Put grated hard cheese (cheddar and/or parmesan) on top of your filling. If your patient is at the stage when he or she can tolerate cheese. If the cheese is not tolerated then you can use home-made mayonnaise instead.

8. Desserts

Baked apples

With a sharp knife scoop out the cores with the seeds from large cooking apples. Fill each apple with a teaspoon of honey a teaspoon of butter, ground or coarsely chopped apricot kernels (or walnuts, or any other available nuts, or desiccated coconut). Add a dried apricot per apple (optional) cut into small pieces. Bake in the oven ati6o-i8o°C (32o-36o°F) for 20-25 minutes.

Crbme-caramel

For one person you need:

3 tablespoons of water 1 teaspoon of honey ground cinnamon

Multiply the ingredients per number of people you want to serve.

Mix all the ingredients well. Pour into shallow ramekin dishes (or any other small terracotta dishes): you need one ramekin dish per person. Sprinkle some cinnamon on top. Preheat the oven to i50°C (300°F). Bake for 30-40 minutes. Apple crumble

4 cooking apples

2 eggs

carrot pulp from juicing 2 lb. of carrots on lb carrots, very finely chopped 10 dried apricots

% a cup ofhoney

% a cup ofunsalted butter

Cut the apples into pieces and place on the bottom of your baking dish. Chop dried apricots into small pieces.

Mix together eggs, butter, carrot pulp, chopped dried apricots and honey. Put the mixture on top of the apples, mix slightly with the apples. Bake in the oven at 150 °C (30o°F) for approximately 40 minutes.

Apple pie
4 large cooking apples
a handful of raisins

ll2 cup of honey

1 cup of fresh or frozen blackcurrants

fresh pumpkin peeled and finely chopped, 2-3 cups pitted dried dates, 2 cups

1 cup of hazelnuts

'l2 cup of ground almonds

Soak the dates in 2 cups of water for 2-3 hours. Drain the dates and reserve. Put the soaking water into your baking dish. Add cored and sliced apples, raisins and blackcurrants. Spread them evenly and sprinkle with the ground almonds. Pour honey on top spreading evenly.

In a food processor blend the dates, pumpkin and hazelnuts. Spoon out this mixture on top of the pie spreading evenly. Slightly press and smooth with a spoon or a knife so that the top looks like the top of a pie. Bake at 150-170°C (300-350T) for an hour.

Winter squash cake

6 eggs

2 cups of grated (packed tightly) winter squash with sweet orange flesh (buttercup, butternut or other)

'/4 a cup of honey

73 cup ofbutter (or ghee, coconutfat, goose fat or duck fat)

3cups of ground almonds 3 medium-size apples

Grease your baking dish and cover the bottom with apples, cored and cut into slices. If your patient's digestive system is sensitive, then peel the apples. Otherwise you can leave the skins on.

Blend the rest of the ingredients in your blender and put the mixture on top of the apples. Smooth the top and bake at i50°C (3oo°F) for 40-50 minutes.

Cake Pinocchio

2 cups of shelled hazelnuts

1 cup of honey (250ml)

4 eggs

50g unsalted butter, preferably organic 4 tangerines to decorate

Preheat the oven to 175-200°C (350-400°F).

Roast the hazelnuts in the oven and rub their skins off. Reserve 1 cup of the nuts for the cream and grind the rest into a coarse flour.

Make 4 circles out of baking paper large enough to fit on a large cake dish and grease them with butter. Separate the whites of the eggs from the yolks. Whip the egg whites stiff with half of the honey. Carefully fold in the ground hazelnuts. Spread the mixture on the four baking paper circles and bake for 5-10 minutes. Cool down and remove the baking paper.

Cream. Soften the butter by leaving it in the room for a few hours.

Whip the 4 egg yolks with the rest of the honey until they increase in volume and become pale whitish in colour. Beat in the butter gradually, adding it in small amounts.

Coarsely chop the rest of the hazelnuts, reserving 10-15 whole nuts for decorating.

Layer the meringue circles with the cream, sprinkling every cream layer with the coarsely chopped hazelnuts. Cover the top with a thin layer of the cream. Peal the tangerines and separate them into segments. Decorate the top with the segments of tangerines and the 10-15 whole hazelnuts. Refrigerate.

Peanut butter pie

6 eggs

2 tablespoons of butter

1 cup of peanut butter

2 cups of carrot pulp left after juicing carrots (you can use winter squash as a substitute, peelit and chop very finely) 'ls cup of honey

1cup of ground almonds

2 large cooking apples

a handful of raisins

Peel the apples, cut them into small pieces and place them into a greased baking dish. Sprinkle the raisins on top of the apples.

In a blender put the rest of the ingredients and blend well. Put the mixture on top of the apples. Smooth the top and bake at 150°C for 40-50 minutes.

Russian custard for one person:

2 eggyolks

%-1 teaspoon of honey

multiply the ingredientsfor the number ofpeople to be served.

Russian Custard can be used instead of cream on fruit or you can serve it on its own with some chopped nuts on the top or pieces of fruit. It can also be used instead of cream in making cakes. Separate the eggyolks from the whites, add the honey and whip the mixture until it goes thick and almost white. As well as being a delicious desert, it provides very good nutrition. Get your eggs from a source you trust. Free range organic eggs are the best.

Apple sauce

5-6 large cooking apples 72 cup butter

1-2 cups water

1-2 cups honey

Peel and core the apples, cut them into pieces and cook in a pan with the water until soft. Take off the heat and add butter. Cool down, mash and sweeten with honey.

You can make pear sauce the same way though you may not need to add honey, as pears are naturally very sweet.

This sauce will keep well in the refrigerator and can be served with some yoghurt, chopped nuts, Russian custard or on its own.

Birthday cake

Make an apple sauce from 5-6 large cooking apples and cool it down. Make it quite sweet as the pastry of the cake is not going to be sweetened. You can make a pear sauce instead of apple.

Separate yolks and whites of 6 eggs into two large bowls. Whip the yolks until thick and light in colour. Whip the whites until firm and no longer runny. Combine the two and add 2 cups of ground almonds. Mix well. Bake in a cake tin lined with greased baking paper for 40 minutes to 1 hour at a temperature of 150°C (300°F). Test with a dry knife whether it is cooked inside (the knife will come out dry if the cake is ready). Depending on the oven the baking time may vary. When ready allow the cake to cool down.

Now the fun part starts. With a long knife cut off the top of the cake making sure that this layer is no more than 1 cm thick. Put it aside for using as the top of your cake later. Using a table spoon carefully spoon out the inside of the cake in medium sized chunks into a separate dish leaving just an outside shell, which will look like a dish ready to be filled. Fill it up with layers of your apple sauce (or pear sauce), frozen raspberries, chopped nuts and chunks of cake, which you spooned out before. Here you can really improvise by using different berries, stoned cherries, pieces of soft fresh fruit, chopped nuts and seeds (sesame, poppy, and sunflower). When the "cake dish" is filled, cover it with the top layer you removed earlier. Spread the remaining apple sauce on and decorate. To decorate you can use fresh fruit, berries, nuts and desiccated coconut. After decorating is done, put the cake into the refrigerator. It is best to make this cake the day before the party so it has the time to "mature" over night.

This is the basic recipe. You can improvise by adding seeds, chopped nuts, grated carrot or pumpkin into the pastry before baking, filling it with different combinations of fruit and berries, and decorating it any way you like. Children like to be involved in decorating. Any of the decorating ingredients, which I have mentioned before, are optional depending on your family's sensitivities. These are fruit, berries, nuts, seeds, fresh mint leaves and coconut.

Ice-cream

Buy in advance some very ripe bananas (with brown spots on the skin), peal them and put in the freezer. On a day when you want to make the ice- cream, get these frozen bananas out and leave them in the room for about 30 minutes to slightly defrost. Blend them in a food processor. Add a little bit of water to make a good creamy consistency. You can blend in some fresh or frozen berries, pieces of fruit, desiccated or fresh coconut to the mixture and some coarsely chopped nuts to make different flavours.

Fresh coconut

When you are buying a coconut, make sure that the shell has no cracks or any other damage to it. Put the nut close to your ear and shake it. If the coconut is healthy, you will hear its juice splashing inside. When a coconut is damaged and its juice has leaked out, then it will be rancid and unsuitable to eat.

When you bring your coconut home, the fun bit starts. You will need a screwdriver and a hammer. At the top of the coconut there are three round dots. Push your screwdriver through 2 of those dots to make 2 holes. Drain the juice through one of the holes allowing the air to get inside through the other hole. The juice is very nourishing and can be used in cooking or drunk as it is. It should have a fresh sweet taste. If the juice tastes rancid, then there is no point in cracking your coconut, it will be unsuitable to eat. After draining the juice crack the shell with the hammer and separate the pulp from the shell. Rinse the pulp with the water to wash off any small bits of shell. There are number of ways to eat it:

• Cut the pulp into small pieces and eat it as it is. It has a very pleasant sweet taste.

• Grind it in your food processor to make sweets (nextrecipe).

• Put the pulp through your juicer to produce a thick coconut cream, which can be diluted with water to make a delicious coconut milk. The cream and milk can be added to your cooking, used as a dressing for fruit and vegetable salads, as a cream for cakes or a replacement for custard.

• Mince the coconut pulp to use in your baking, home made ice-cream and other desserts, soups, stews, salads and sauces.

A word of caution for children and adults with diarrhoea. Coconut is very fibrous and may make the diarrhoea worse, so initially I suggest putting the coconut through a juicer, which would separate the fibre from the rest of it. This way you can enjoy the freshly made coconut milk and cream, getting all the good nutrition from them without the fibre.

Coconut sweets

1 medium-size coconut

1 cup of dried fruit (can be any of the following: dried apricots, figs, dates or raisins, or a mixture of them. Make sure they are not sorbated or coated in starch)

1 cup of sesame seeds or ground almonds

Soak the dried fruit for 6-8 hours. Drain.

Make two holes in the coconut and drain the liquid. Put the liquid through a fine sieve and reserve for the recipe.

Shell the coconut and rinse the pulp to wash away small bits of shell. Cut the coconut pulp into pieces small enough to put through your grinder or juicer.

Grind the coconut pulp with the dried fruit. Mix well in your food pro- cessor or by hand. If the mixture is too dry, add some liquid from the coconut, which you have reserved.

With your hands roll small balls from the mixture and coat them in sesame seeds or ground almonds. Place on a large plate and refrigerate.

9. Egg-freerecipes

Eggs are used in baking as a binder to keep all the other ingredients together. Some children have a true allergy to eggs and have to avoid them. The following ingredients will act as a binder in your baking instead of eggs.

• Gelatine, well dissolved in a small amount of hot water;

• Pumpkin, baked and mashed;

• Butternut squash and other winter squashes (acorn, turban, hubbard, spaghetti), baked and mashed;

• Banana, mashed;

• Apple, baked and mashed or made into an apple souse;

• Pear, baked and mashed or made into a sauce;

• Zucchini (marrow or courgettes), baked, mashed and drained of excess liquid.

Egg-free hreadlcake/muffin mixture

2 cups of ground nuts (almonds, cashews, walnuts, hazels, etc.)

3 tablespoons of butter (or coconut oil, ghee, goose fat, duck fat)

2 cups of cooked and mashed squash (butternut squash, pumpkin or other less watery squashes, apple sauce, pear sauce)

To prepare the squash (pumpkin), cut it into two halves and remove the seeds. Place on a baking tray with the cut surface down and bake in the oven until very soft (a knife should go through it very easily). Cool, scoop out all the inside and mash with a fork.

You can improvise on this recipe by adding to the mixture honey, dried fruit, coarsely chopped nuts, shredded coconut, berries and fruit pieces.

Mix all the ingredients well. Put into a well-buttered baking dish and bake in the oven at 150-175°C (300~350°F) for 45 minutes to an hour. Occasionally check with a dry knife if it is ready (the knife has to come out dry).

If in the same mixture you add 2 tablespoons of pure tomato puree (with a single ingredient: tomato), some salt and pepper, you can bake a pizza base. Just spread the mixture on a baking paper, shaping it with a spoon.

Experiment with your own varieties, using ingredients available to you from the allowed list. Here are a few examples of egg-free recipes you can make.

Egg free-banana muffins

2 cups of cashew nuts or any other nuts

2 ripe bananas

4 teaspoons of honey

4 teaspoons of gelatine powder or crystals 4-8 tablespoons of coconut oil or butter

Grind the nuts into a flour (you can use ground almonds instead). Mash the banana. Dissolve gelatine powder in half a cup of hot water.

Mix all the ingredients together. Fill paper muffin cases with the mixture and bake at 150-170°C (380°F) for 15-20 minutes.

You can vary this recipe by folding in different berries into the mixture, small pieces of fruit, coarsely chopped nuts or seeds (sunflower, sesame or pumpkin).

Egg-free Easter Eggs

2 cups of pecans

a handful of coconut flakes

4 tablespoons of butter or ghee 2 tablespoons of honey

Blend all the ingredient in the food processor into a fine paste. With your hands roll out small eggs. Put them in the freezer until ready to eat.

With this mixture you can make different biscuits, using children's biscuit shapes. Roll the mixture on a well-buttered surface until 1 cm thick. Put it into a freezer for 2 hours or longer, take out and cut into shapes (squares, animals, tractors, etc.). You can let your children do the cutting out.

Egg-free crackers/biscuits

2 tablespoons of butter (coconut oil or duck fat/goose fat)

2 cups of ground nuts (almonds, hazels, walnuts, etc.)

2-3 tablespoons of water (or almond milk or coconut milk)

You can improvise by adding to this mixture herbs, cinnamon, paprika, cayenne pepper, black pepper, salt, grated cheddar cheese (if well toler- ated) or peanut butter.

Mix the ingredients well. Roll out thinly on a board, sprinkled with some ground nuts. Cut into squares or any other shapes. Sprinkle some coarse salt, poppyseeds, caraway seeds or coriander seeds on top. Bake in the oven on well-buttered baking paper ati50°C (300°F) for 10-15 minutes.

Egg-free fruit dessert

1. Blend or cut into small pieces available berries and fruit and cover the bottom of your baking tin with the mixture. Nice combinations are plums and apples, pears and raspberries, cherries and pineapple, apple and blackcurrants.

2. Pour about 3 cups of ground almonds over the fruit.

3. Sprinkle \k cups of shredded coconut over the almonds.

4. Spread 1-2 cups of pecan halves over the coconut (you can use any other available nuts, coarsely chopped).

5. Cover the top with 200g of butter, cut into slices (you can use coconut oil or ghee instead of butter).

6. Bake ati6o-i75°C (350°F) for about 40 minutes.

Egg-free apple pie

1. Fill your baking dish halfway up with peeled and chopped cooking apples and plums (take the stones out). Instead of plums you can use blackcurrants, raspberries, blackberries, pears, elderberries, etc.

2. Pour half a cup of honey over the fruit and mix lightly.

3. Soak two handfuls of dried dates in half a cup of hot water to make them softer. Drain and use for the crust. The soaking water is very sweet and can be poured over the fruit.

4. To make the crust blend the dates with 1 cup of ground almonds and 2 tablespoons of butter. With your hands shape the mixture into a bail, put it on a large sheet of baking paper or cling film and roll it out into a round pancake shape large enough to cover the top of your baking dish. Lift up the baking paper with the rolled out pastry and carefully flip it over the fruit. Make sure that the pastry covers the whole of the fruit, trim off any excess and fill any holes with it.

5. Bake in the oven at i3o-i50°C (300°F) for about 40-50 minutes. Egg-free cookies (biscuits)

2 cups of ground nuts (nut flour)

1 cup of cooked and mashed butternut squash pear sauce made from 1 large pear

1 tablespoon of butter or any other acceptable fat

Mix all the ingredients well and bake small biscuits on baking paper at 150- i6o°C (300°F) for about 20 minutes.

10. Beverages

Nut/seed milk

You can use almonds, sunflower seeds, sesame seeds, pine nuts, etc. to make milk. Almonds make the best milk. You can add a teaspoon of flaxseeds to make the milk thicker. Soak the nuts/seeds in water for 12-24 hours, drain. Blend in a food processor with water: fori cup of nuts/seeds add 2-3 cups of water. A good juicer will crush the nuts/seeds well, making a paste, which you blend with water. Mix well and strain through a cheese-cloth or a fine strainer and you have got milk. You can add some soaked dates or raisins, when blending, they will make the milk sweet. If you find that the milk is too rich, just add more water. You can add some freshly pressed apple juice or carrot juice into it to make a very tasty and nourishing drink.

Coconut milk

Bring to boil 1 cup of unsweetened shredded coconut and 1 cup of water. Cool down and blend well in the food processor. Strain through a cheese- cloth or a fine strainer.

Ginger tea

1 tablespoon of freshly grated ginger root water

In your teapot put the grated ginger root and pour over boiling water. Cover and brew for 5-10 minutes. Pore through a sieve. It is a warming drink and aids digestion.

Freshly squeezed juices

Use only organic fruit and vegetables for making juices. Wash your fruit and vegetables and cut any bad bits off. Do not peel and do not remove seeds.

A good juice to start the day is pineapple + carrot + small amount of beetroot.

The most therapeutic juices do not taste very nice: green and vegetable juices. To make your juices tasty and enjoyable to drink I recommend making mixes of different fruit and vegetables. You can make all sorts of juice mixes, but generally try to have:

• 50% of highly therapeutic ingredients: carrot, small amount of beet- root (no more than 5% of the juice mixture), celery, white and red cabbage, lettuce, greens (spinach, parsley, dill, basil, fresh nettle leaves, beet tops and carrot tops),

• 50% of some tasty ingredients to disguise the taste of therapeutic ingredients: pineapple, apple, orange, grapefruit, grapes, mango, etc.

Your patient can have these juices as they are or diluted with some water. If throughout the day your GAPS child would not drink just water, you can add some of these freshly squeezed juices into the water to make a tasty drink. Initially start with 1 cup of juice a day. With a small child you may want to start from a very small amount, like 1 teaspoon a day. Increase the daily amount very gradually until your child has 2 cups of freshly squeezed juices a day. These juices should be taken on an empty stomach, so first thing in the morning and middle of the afternoon are good times.

With these juices you can make ice-lollies. Just fill ice-lolly forms with freshly squeezed juice and freeze.

You can also make ice-cubes from these juices which can be used to make a cold drink in hot weather. Just fill the glass with these ice-cubes and add mineral water (still or carbonated).

The carrot pulp left from juicing can be used in your baking mixtures together with ground nuts or as a replacement for ground nuts. You can also use pulp left from other fruit and vegetables depending on your taste preferences.

Fruit smoothies

You can make all sorts of combinations. If you make your own goat's yoghurt, then you can use it as well. Here are a few ideas.

Blend a banana with 72 ripe avocado, half a cup of home-made goat's yoghurt and a bit of honey to taste.

Half an avocado blended with freshly squeezed apple/carrot juice or freshly squeezed pineapple juice.

Banana blended with freshly squeezed carrot juice (apple juice, pine- apple juice, orange juice, etc.) and half a cup of yoghurt.

11. Yoghurt and creme fraiche

In the initial stages many GAPS patients tolerate goat's yoghurt better than cow's. So, try to make yoghurt from goat's milk first. I strongly recommend using only organic milk. A lot of milk on the supermarket shelves has been subjected to a process, called homogenisation in order to stop milk from separating in the bottle. This process breaks down the fat globules and changes the structure of milk making it harmful for the body. Try to buy milk, which apart from pasteurisation, has not been subjected to any processing.

Goat's yoghurt is quite a lot more liquid than cow's yoghurt. You can use it as a drink or if you want to thicken it you can drip it through cheese- cloth.

To make yoghurt you need to introduce bacteria into the milk. You can buy commercially available yoghurt starters from many health food shops or small-holding suppliers. Alternatively you can use commercially avail- able live yoghurt as a starter. After making their first yoghurt many people successfully perpetuate their own yoghurt by using it as a starter for the next batch. You can also keep the liquid left from dripping your yoghurt in a clean dry jar in your refrigerator to use as a starter for making the next batch of yoghurt. If at any point your own yoghurt or the "dripping liquid" do not work you need to start again with a commercial starter or commer- cial live yoghurt.

Instructions for making yoghurt

1. In a stainless steal pan bring close to the boil I litre of milk (goat's or cow's) stirring occasionally. You need to bring the milk close to boiling point in order to destroy any bacteria, which may linger in the milk and interfere with the fermentation. However, do not boil the milk, as it will change its taste. Take the pan off the heat. Cover the pan with the lid and cool down by placing the pan into cold water until the temperature of the milk is around 38-45°C. If you do not have a suitable thermometer use your own hand to determine the right temperature. To do that take a teaspoon of milk from the pan (using a clean dry spoon) and put the milk on the inside of your wrist. If it feels just slightly warm then the temperature is right.

2. If you are using a commercial yoghurt starter in a powder form you need to dissolve the powder in a little milk first before adding it to the pan. If you are using your own yoghurt or commercial live yoghurt add 7a cup into the milk. Stir well, cover with the lid and put in a warm place preferably at 38-45°C. You can use a clean dry thermos for this purpose, a yoghurt maker, an electric plate, the top of your boiler or your airing cabinet (if it is warm enough). Ferment the yoghurt for at least 24 hours or longer.

3. After the fermentation is complete, move the yoghurt into a clean dry glass jar, cover and refrigerate.

4. To drip the yoghurt line a large colander with a cheese-cloth. Place the colander into alarge bowl and pouryour yoghurt into the lined colander. Cover with a tea towel and let it drip for a few hours. You can collect the liquid after dripping and keep it refrigerated in a dry glass jar to re-use as

a starter. You can also use this liquid for soaking the liver in to remove any bitter taste before cooking it. Depending on how long you leave your yoghurt dripping you can make a soft cottage cheese or thicker yoghurt. Both soft cottage cheese and the yoghurt can be used for baking, adding to salads and soups and as desserts with honey and fruit.

Instructions for making creme fraiche

By using cream instead of milk you can make creme fraiche or soured cream. For llitre of cream use one sachet of commercial starter or I cup of live yoghurt.

1. Constantly stirring, bring the cream to boil but do not let it boil.

2. Cool down by placing the pan into cold water. Keep the pan covered at all times.

3. Test the temperature, it should be 38-45°C.

4. Add the starter and ferment for 24 hours minimum.

This soured cream or creme fraiche is very nice to use in salads, soups, stews, in baking or as a dessert with some honey and berries. You can blend it with a little honey and frozen fruit or berries to make an instant ice- cream.